Nursing Procedures

Volume 1: Venipuncture, Intravenous Line, Blood Transfusion and Injection Procedures

Solomon Barroa, R.N.

Copyright 2013

All rights reserved. No part of this book may be reproduced by any means, electronic, mechanical, photocopying, recording, scanning or otherwise without permission from the author. The author reserves the right not to be responsible for the correctness, completeness or quality of the information provided. Liability claims regarding damage caused by the use of any information provided, including any kind of information that is incomplete or incorrect, will be rejected. The information contained in this book does not constitute medical advice, and is for information and educational purposes only. Consult your health care provider regarding health concerns.

To Dr. Lee Robbins, Mary Ann, Rosario, Vicente, Benedicto, and Robert.

Introduction and Purpose

Nursing is a profession devoted to compassionate care and assisting an individual to recover from a disease or a body condition. The success of the nursing profession relies mostly on three factors: the nurse, the client and technology. A nurse who has earned training, skills and licensure is expected to be knowledgeable and skillful about implementing a procedure ordered by a physician. The client who receives care can favorably affect the outcome of the nursing care through compliance, cooperation and feedback. Use of technology requires quality and appropriateness. These three factors interact resulting in either a successful outcome or the worsening of a client's condition.

The ultimate goal of the nursing procedure is to help in the diagnosis and treatment. It is an inseparable component of the nursing care plan and the implementation process. Nursing procedures are dependent on the skills and knowledge of the nurse, the technology being used and the client's compliance, cooperation and feedback. The success of the nursing procedure and its applicability can be predictable by the nurse even before implementation. There are nursing procedures questionable for applicability and foreseeable outcome. Using nursing procedures for the purpose of diagnosis is helpful in preventing the worsening of a bodily condition. The majority of diagnostic procedures require blood testing with the results analyzed in the laboratory. There are hundreds of nursing procedures that a nurse should know, and more of these procedures are continually created as new technologies are implemented in the field of healthcare. Research has shown that majority of these nursing procedures are never performed by an individual nurse due to the many divisions of the nursing profession. A nurse who works in a geriatric clinic may never participate in cardiac catheterization or a utilization review nurse may never perform an OASIS assessment. In the ever changing and dynamic provision of healthcare, a nurse may attain practice experience or continuing education in some nursing procedures that he or she has never performed.

This volume series presents medical information to nurses and allied healthcare professionals who are continuously implementing various nursing procedures. Techniques in implementing nursing procedures may vary from one institution to another. It is up to the discretion of the reader to follow the institutional policies for implementing the different nursing procedures presented in this volume series. There are short tests and quizzes located at the end of every chapter. The author disclaims any responsibility for the correctness and applicability of the various materials presented. The contents were acquired through rigorous research and are not intended to substitute for the knowledge and skills of the reader. This volume series is intended for educational purposes and does not constitute medical advisement or substitution.

For questions and comments, the author can be reached at:

solomon_barroa@yahoo.com

and at: http://www.amazon.com/Solomon-Barroa-RN/e/B00AV3V34S

Thank you for buying this book. I hope that it caused satisfaction and happiness.

Table Of Contents

Chapter 1 Overview of the Cardiovascular, Integumentary and Muscular Systems 6
Chapter 1 Test (Overview of the Anatomy and Physiology) *11*

Chapter 2 Venipuncture 16
Chapter 2 Test (Venipuncture) *19*

Chapter 3 Intravenous Line 21
Chapter 3 Test (IV Line) *25*

Chapter 4 Blood Transfusion 27
Chapter 4 Test (Blood Transfusion) *30*

Chapter 5 Intradermal Injection 31
Chapter 5 Test (Intradermal Injection) *33*

Chapter 6 Subcutaneous Injection 34
Chapter 6 Test (Subcutaneous Injection) *37*

Chapter 7 Intramuscular Injection 38
Chapter 7 Test (Intramuscular Injection) *41*

Answer Key 43

References 51

Index 52

Chapter 1 Overview of the Cardiovascular, Integumentary and Muscular Systems

The cardiovascular system comprises the heart, blood vessels and blood. These organs function to provide oxygenated blood to the whole body and maintain tissue perfusion. The heart is a muscular organ that pumps blood to the body. It has three layers; pericardium, myocardium and endocardium. The pericardium is the outer layer, myocardium the middle and endocardium the innermost layer. The heart is composed of four chambers; right and left atriums and right and left ventricles. The right and left atriums are upper chambers while the right and left ventricles are lower chambers. Flaps of valve called tricuspid separate the right atrium from the right ventricle. The left atrium and left ventricle are separated by flaps of valves called mitral. The heart is connected to the lungs through the pulmonary vein and artery. The pulmonary vein carries the oxygenated blood from the lungs while the pulmonary artery carries the deoxygenated blood toward the lungs. The heart's rhythm and heartbeat is initiated by electrical impulses that originate from the sinoatrial node (known as pacemaker).

Blood with a low oxygen level from the various parts of the body goes to the heart through the venae cavae. The venae cavae are the largest veins in the body. It is composed of two branches, superior and inferior vena cava. The blood from the upper part of the body flows to the superior vena cava while blood from the lower part of the body flows to the inferior vena cava. The bloods from the venae cavae enter the heart through the right atrium. Next, it passes the tricuspid valve to the right ventricle. From there, the blood is pumped out. It passes the pulmonary valve to the pulmonary artery and into the lungs. This is where the low oxygen level blood obtains oxygen through the exchange of gases in the capillaries. The air sacs of the lungs are connected to the capillaries. Diffusion enables exchange of the gases carbon dioxide and oxygen. After the blood gets oxygenated, it travels back to the heart through the pulmonary vein and into the left atrium. It then passes the mitral valve to the left ventricle. From the left ventricle, the oxygenated blood is pumped to the aortic valve and into the aorta to be distributed to the different parts of the body.

The blood vessels are comprised of the veins, arteries and capillaries. Vena cava is the largest vein in the human body. It is composed of the inferior and superior vena cavae that carry unoxygenated blood from the different parts of the body into the right atrium of the heart. The veins of the circulatory system carry deoxygenated blood from the different parts of the body. They transport blood to the heart.

The blood is oxygenated in the lungs after passing through the right side of the heart. The pulmonary vein is the only vein that carries oxygenated blood from the lungs. The larger veins in the body branch into smaller ones called venules. These venules connect to capillaries. The capillaries, microscopic in size, function for exchanging body nutrients and wastes. This is also where the blood is oxygenated. The blood travels to the arterioles after it has been oxygenated. The arterioles are small branches of arteries that connect to the big arteries. The aorta is the largest artery in the human body. It carries oxygenated blood. The constriction and dilation of the blood vessels is known to directly affect blood pressure.

The pressure produced by the circulating blood upon the walls of the blood vessel is called the blood pressure. It is also known as the arterial pressure. It is subdivided into two specific types. These are the systolic and diastolic pressures. The systolic pressure is the highest pressure in the arteries. It occurs when the heart contracts and the blood is ejected into the aorta and the arteries. It is the upper number in a blood pressure measurement. The diastolic pressure is the lowest pressure and occurs when the heart is relaxed. The blood returns to the heart from the vena cava and the veins. It is the lower number in a blood pressure measurement.

The blood system is composed of cells such as RBC (red blood cell), WBC (white blood cell) and platelets. RBC is also known as erythrocyte. WBC is composed of agranulocytes, granulocytes and leukocytes. Agranulocytes are white blood cells with one large nucleus. They are composed of lymphocytes and monocytes. Lymphocyte is a type of white blood cell with a large dark stainable nucleus. Lymphocytes produce antibodies. Monocytes are formed in the bone marrow. They become macrophages after leaving the blood and function for phagocytosis. Granulocytes are white blood cells with multiple granules. They are composed of basophils, eosinophils and neutrophils. Basophils are characterized by large and dark granules. Eosinophils have a dense and reddish granule. Neutrophils have a neutral staining granule. They are produced in the bone marrow and function for phagocytosis. Leukocytes are another type of white blood cells that fights infectious agents. A platelet cell is also known as thrombocyte.

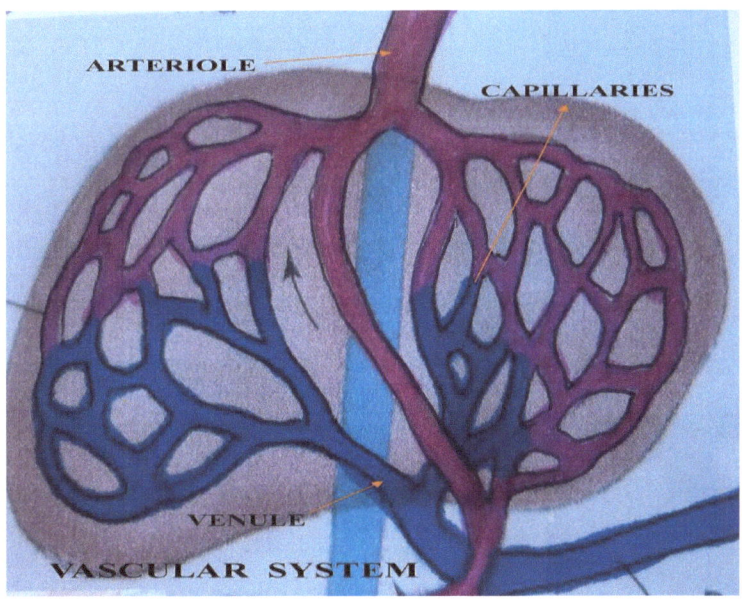

The blood is a liquid medium from which all chemical substances are transported throughout the body including foreign agents such as bacteria and parasites. It carries waste products such as urea and ammonia towards the kidney to be eliminated and carries nutrients from the intestines to the cells of the different organs of the body. The nutrients that the blood carries are albumin (protein), glucose (carbohydrate) and lipids (fats). Through the blood, gases such as oxygen maintain the perfusion of all the different systems in the body. Electrolytes such as sodium and potassium are also transported, eliminated and reabsorbed.

There are four blood types. These are types A, B, AB and O. These blood types contain different antigens and antibodies. An antigen is a foreign entity that triggers the production of antibodies. These antibodies are protein substances that neutralize an antigen. The blood type AB is considered a universal receiver because it can receive blood from all other blood types. This blood type cannot donate to blood types A and B because of its antigens. Blood type O is known as the universal donor because it can be donated to all blood types but can only receive blood of its own type. The blood type B can receive blood from types B and O but can only donate to types AB and B. Blood type A can receive blood from types A and O but can only donate to types AB and A.

In the process of blood transfusion, a mismatch between blood types will trigger an antibody and antigen reaction. This reaction results in agglutination or the clumping of a recipient's blood. It produces an acute hemolytic reaction through the destruction of erythrocytes. Symptoms such as fever, chills, chest pain, shortness of breath and sudden drops in blood pressure occur. The initial intervention will be to immediately stop the transfusion.

The formation of a blood clot is important when there is a wound because it promotes healing and formation of a new skin. It is a process that stops the loss of blood from a damaged blood vessel. Blood clotting is also known as coagulation or thrombogenesis. This process is complex and requires different substances and chemical reactions. Initially the circulating platelets react to bind with collagen through glycoprotein receptors. Adhesion is started through this process. Blood factors for clotting such as the von Willebrand factor, are then released to further strengthen the adhesion. Calcium will be released in the platelets through the chemical changes brought about by the clotting factors. From these, the prothrombinase enzyme will be released. It converts prothrombin protein to an enzyme called thrombin. The enzyme thrombin will then convert the protein fibrinogen to fibrin. Finally fibrin forms the threads of clots.

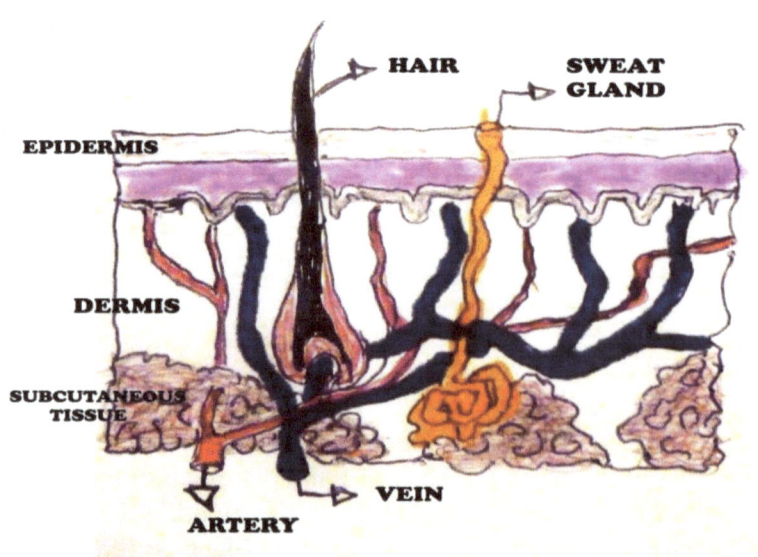

Layers and Structures of the Skin

The skin is called the integumentary system. It covers and protects the human body. It also provides color and identity. The healthy skin is usually smooth and free from bumps. Hairs and nails are appendages of the integumentary system. There are three layers of the skin; epidermis, dermis and hypodermis. The epidermis is the outermost layer that is composed of 5 strata (sub layers); stratum corneum, lucidum, granulosum, spinosum and basale. The main functions of the epidermis are hydration, providing color and a barrier to the surrounding environment. Skin color is due to the pigment melanin. Dermis is the second layer of the skin that is composed of 2 strata, papillare and reticulare. It contains nerve receptors, sweat glands, hair follicles, lymphatic and blood vessels. The hypodermis is the third layer of the skin. It is mostly composed of fat cells.

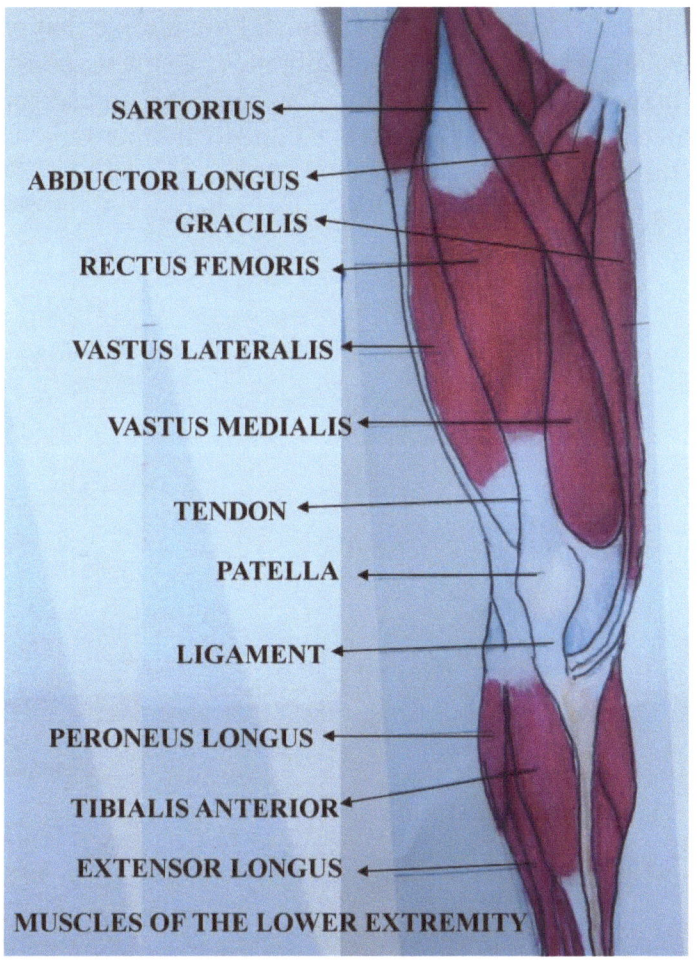

Muscles are soft tissues that produce force and motion. There are 3 types of muscles; skeletal, cardiac and smooth. Skeletal muscles are voluntary muscles that are anchored by tendons to a bone. Cardiac muscles are involuntary muscles found in the heart. Smooth muscles are involuntary muscles that are found within the walls of body organs such as the stomach, intestines, blood vessels, uterus, urethra and urinary bladder. The movement of muscles (contractions) is stimulated by the electrical impulses of the motor nerves (motor neurons).

The different types of movement are abduction, adduction, dorsiflexion, extension, flexion, plantar flexion, pronation, rotation and supination. Abduction is a movement away from the midline plane of the body such as reaching for things. Adduction is a movement toward the midline plane of the body such as moving the knees to touch each other. Dorsiflexion is a movement where the foot is brought upward closer to the shin. Extension is a movement of increasing the angle between two surfaces such as straightening the limbs of the body. Flexion is a movement that decreases the angle between two surfaces such as bending a limb of the body. Plantar flexion is a movement that extends the foot downwards. Pronation is a movement where the palm is turned backward and down. Rotation is a circular movement around an axis such as rotating the arms. Supination is a movement where the palm is turned forward and up.

There are special structures of the neuromuscular system such as bursa, fascia, ligaments and tendons. Bursa is a fluid filled sac that is lined by a synovial membrane that provides cushioning between muscles and bones in a joint. A synovial membrane is a soft tissue found in joints. Fascia is a fibrinous membrane or a connective tissue that separates and surrounds muscles. Ligament is a fibrous connective tissue that connects a bone to another bone in the body. Tendon is a fibrous connective tissue that connects a muscle to a bone.

Chapter 1 Test (Overview of the Anatomy and Physiology)

The Muscular System

I. Multiple Choice Choose the best answer/s from the following statements. There could be one or more answer/s from the selection.

1. Abduction is a movement (a. away b. toward c. sideways d. into) from the midline plane of the body.

2. Adduction is a movement (a. away b. toward c. side d. from) the midline plane of the body.

3. Dorsiflexion is a movement where the foot is brought (a. away b. sideways c. closer d. distal) to the shin upward.

4. (a. Flexion b. Pronation c. Supination d. Extension) is a movement increasing the angle between two surfaces such as straightening the limbs of the body.

5. (a. Flexion b. Extension c. Supination d. Pronation) is a movement that decreases the angle between two surfaces such as bending inward a limb of the body.

6. (a. Dorsiflexion b. Plantar flexion c. Pronation d. Supination) is a movement that extends the foot downwards.

7. Pronation is a movement where the palm is turned (a. sideways b. forward c. backward d. upward) and down.

8. Rotation is when there is (a. angular b. pivotal c. perpendicular d. circular) movement around an axis.

9. Supination = is a movement where the palm is turned (a. forward b. backward c. sideways d. circular) and up.

11

10. (a. Tendon b. Ligament c. Bursa d. Fascia) is a fibrous connective tissue that connects a bone to another bone in the body.

11. (a. Ligament b. Bursa c. Tendon d. Fascia) is a fibrous connective tissue that connects a muscle to a bone.

12. (a. Fascia b. Synovia c. Patella d. Bursa) is a fluid filled sac that is lined by a synovial membrane, which provides cushioning between muscles and bones in a joint.

13. (a. Fascia b. Ligament c. Tendon d. Cartilage) is a fibrous membrane or a connective tissue that separates and surrounds muscles.

14. The striated muscle is also called (a. smooth b. skeletal c. involuntary d. striated smooth) muscle.

15. The smooth muscle is also called (a. voluntary b. striated c. visceral d. smooth) muscle.

The Cardiovascular System

I. Multiple Choice.   Choose the best answer/s from the following statements. There could be one or more answer/s from the selection.

1. The (a. right ventricle b. tricuspid valve c. left atrium d. right atrium) is the upper chamber of the heart where the blood enters.

2. The (a. left atrium b. ventricle c. atrium d. right atrium) is the lower chamber of the heart where the blood is collected and pushed out.

3. The (a. bicuspid b. mitral c. tricuspid d. atrial) valve is located between the right atrium and right ventricle. It is also called the right atrioventricular valve.

4. The (a. pulmonary b. b. bicuspid c. mitral d. tricuspid) valve is located between the right ventricle and pulmonary artery.

5. The (a. pulmonic b. tricuspid c. aortic d. mitral valve) is located between the left atrium and the left ventricle. It is also called the left atrioventricular valve.

6. The (a. pulmonic b. aortic c. mitral d. tricuspid) valve is located between the left ventricle and the aorta.

7. The (a. pericardium b. endocardium c. myocardium d. mesocardium) is the middle layer of the heart consisting of cardiac muscles.

8. The (a. pericardium b. ectocardium c. parietal membrane d. myocardium) is the outermost layer consisting of double layered membrane that covers the heart.

9. The (a. atrioventricular node b. purkinje fibers c. bundle of His d. sinoatrial node) is a tissue that generates impulses. It is located in the right atrium of the heart.

10. The (a. sinoatrial node b. atrioventricular node c. purkinje fibers d. bundle of His) is a tissue that coordinate impulses between the atrium and the ventricle. It is located between the atria and ventricles of the heart.

11. The (sinoatrial node b. atrioventricular node c. Bundle of His d. purkinje fibers) is tissue that transmits impulses from the atrioventricular node to the Purkinje fibers.

12. The (a. Purkinje fiber b. sinoatrial node c. atrioventricular node d. right and left bundle of His) generates electrical impulses to the ventricle. It is located in the inner ventricular walls of the heart.

13. (a. Systole b. Ventricular dilation c. Asystole d. Diastole) is a period when the heart refills with blood and when the ventricles are relaxing.

14. (a. Diastole b. Systole c. Ventricular diastole d. Atrial diastole) is a period when the ventricle of the heart is contracting.

15. (a. Vasodilation b. Stenosis c. Vasoconstriction d. Sclerosis) = is the narrowing of a blood vessel due to the contraction of its muscles.

Hematological System

I. Matching type. Match selection A with selection B with the appropriate word/s. There could be one or more answer/s from the selection

Selection A

_____ 1. Blood type AB
_____ 2. Blood type
_____ 3. Blood type B
_____ 4. Blood type A

Selection B

a. universal donor
b. donates to AB & B
c. universal recipient
d. cannot donate to A & B
e. donates to AB & A
f. receives from A & O
g. receives from B & O

II. Multiple Choice. Choose the appropriate word/s to complete the following statements. There could be one or more answer/s from the selection.

1. (a. Agranulocytes b. Lymphocytes c. Monocytes d. Granulocytes) are white blood cells with one large nucleus. They compose the lymphocytes and monocytes.

2. (a. Erythrocyte b. Hemoglobin c. Hematocrit d. Thrombocyte) is a red blood cell.

3. (a. Agranulocytes b. Granulocytes c. Monocyte d. Lymphocyte) are white blood cells with multiple granules. They are composed of basophils, eosinophils and neutrophils.

4. (a. Thrombocyte b. Leukocyte c. Erythrocyte d. Hematocrit) is a white blood cell.

5. (a. Leukocyte b. Hematocrit c. Erythrocyte d. Thrombocyte) is a platelet cell.

6. (a. Basophil   b. Monocyte   c. Lymphocyte   d. Eosinophil) is a type of white blood cell with large and dark granules.

7. (a. Basophil   b. Monocyte   c. Eosinophil   d. Lymphocyte) is a type of white blood cell with dense and reddish granules.

8. (a. Monocyte   b. Basophil   c. Lymphocyte   d. Neutrophil) is a type of white blood cell with large dark staining nucleus. It produces antibodies.

9. (a. Neutrophil   b. Basophil   c. Lymphocyte   d. Monocyte) is a type of white blood cell that is formed in the bone marrow. It becomes a macrophage after leaving the blood. It functions for phagocytosis.

10. (a. Neutrophil   b. Basophil   c. Eosinophil   d. Monocyte) = is a type of white blood cell with neutral staining granules. It is produced in the bone marrow and functions for phagocytosis.

Chapter 2 Venipuncture

Venipuncture is a procedure used to obtain a blood sample for diagnostic studies and in evaluating the blood structure of an individual. A blood sample is drawn from the veins comprised of venous blood. It is typically performed in the antecubital fossa and veins in the dorsal forearm and dorsum of the hand or foot. The most common veins used for venipuncture are cephalic, basilic and median veins.

Equipment/Materials

Tourniquet
Gloves
Alcohol pads/antiseptic swabs
Syringe or evacuated tubes/Vacutainer tubes
20/21 gauge needle for adults or 23/25 gauge for children
Color coded collection tubes
Labels
Sterile 2 x 2 gauze pads
Adhesive bandage or tape

Preparing evacuated/Vacutainer tubes require opening the needle packet, attaching the double ended needle to its holder and selecting the appropriate tube. The long end of the needle is used to puncture the vein while the short end fits into the collection tube. Preparing the syringe requires attaching the appropriate needle. Label all collection tubes.

Procedure

1. Wash hands and apply gloves.

2. Explain procedure to the client and inquire if there was untoward reaction such as nausea and fainting during the last venipuncture experience.

3. Assist the ambulatory client to sit on a chair with armrest support for the venipuncture site if using the forearm.

4. Assess the veins of the site and palpate for a firm rebound sensation.
***Avoid collecting blood sample from an infected, injured and edematous site. Using the legs for venipuncture may predispose the client to thrombophlebitis and infection.

5. Tie the tourniquet 5 to 10 cm (2 to 4 inches) above the area chosen to make the veins dilate.
***Tourniquet may be optional for a client with large, distended and highly visible veins to prevent the occurrence of hematoma.

6. Palpate brachial pulse.
***Tight tourniquet impedes arterial blood flow.

7. Clean the site with the alcohol pad in circulation motion from inner to outer. Let it dry.
***Alcohol causes hemolysis of the blood sample if left damp.

8. Immobilize the vein by pressing an inch just below the site using the thumb. Draw the skin taut.
***Immobilizing the vein promotes stability and prevents it from moving during needle insertion.

9. Position the syringe or needle holder at 15 to 30 degree angle with the bevel of needle in the upward position.
***The bevel of the needle in the upward position prevents trauma to the vein.

10. Insert the needle into the vein. Ask the client to close his fist loosely as the needle is inserted and open the fist as soon as the needle is in the vein.

11a. Draw the blood slowly by pulling the plunger of the syringe in a gentle fashion to create a steady suction.
***Forcibly pulling the plunger may collapse the vein.

11b. An evacuated/Vacutainer tube requires grasping the holder securely and pushing down on the collection tube until the needle punctures the rubber stopper and blood flows into the tube automatically.

12. Remove the tourniquet as soon as the blood flows adequately.
***Tourniquet should be removed after 1 to 2 minutes to prevent stasis, localized acidemia and hemoconcentration.

13. Continue collecting blood sample until the tube is filled with the required amount.

14. Remove and insert another tube if needed. Gently rotate or invert tubes with additives to mix it.

15a. Place the gauze pad over the puncture site while slowly and gradually removing the needle from the vein.

15b. When using an evacuated tube, remove the evacuated tube from the needle holder to release the vacuum before withdrawing the needle from the vein.

16. Apply gentle pressure or asks the client to do so at the venipuncture site to prevent the occurrence of hematoma.
***Maintain firm pressure at least 5 minutes for clients with clotting disorders and those on anticoagulant therapy.

17. Apply an adhesive bandage after the bleeding stops.

18. Transfer the blood sample from the syringe to a collection tube gently to avoid foaming and hemoconcentration. Insert the needle through the stopper of the tube and allow vacuum to fill the tube or remove needle and stopper from syringe and gently inject blood to the tube then reapply the tube stopper.
***Forcing blood into the tube causes hemolysis.

19. Gently rotate blood tubes with additives at least 8 to 10 times. Additives prevent blood clot formation.
***Shaking the tube will cause hemolysis of red blood cells.

20. Assess the client for any untoward reaction.
***If client becomes dizzy or faint, position with the head lowered between knees.

21. Discard needles or sharps, gloves and other materials in appropriate containers.

22. Recheck labels and correct identification to prevent errors.

23. Place all collected specimen in a bag to be sent to the laboratory.

The most common complications from the venipuncture site are hematoma and infection. Even the most skilled person may cause such complications. Infection usually results from poor aseptic technique and hematoma due to extravasation. Most institutions delegate venipuncture to phlebotomists who are trained in collecting blood specimen. The nurse may supervise and delegate blood collection as needed.

There are certain requirements for some specimen collection such as those in cryoglobulin levels, ammonia levels, lactic acid levels and vitamin levels. Test tubes are pre-warmed when collecting blood specimen for cryoglobulin levels. Icing the test tube before delivery to the laboratory is a requirement for obtaining a specimen for ammonia levels. Tourniquet is never used in collecting blood samples for lactic acid levels. Test tubes are not exposed to light after obtaining blood samples for vitamin levels.

Chapter 2 Test (Venipuncture)

I. Multiple Choice
Choose the best answer from the following statements.

1. Tight tourniquet impedes (a.arterial b.venous c.capillary d.none of the above) blood flow.

2. Alcohol causes (a.viscosity b.hemolysis c.hemoconcentration d.none of the above) of the blood sample if left damp.

3. The bevel of the needle is in the upward position to prevent (a.trauma b.getting in c.hitting d.none of the above) to the vein.

4. Forcibly pulling the plunger of the syringe may (a.hit b.collapse c.puncture d.none of the above) the vein.

5-6. Tourniquet should be removed after (a.3 to 4 b.3 to 5 c.1 to 2 d.2 to 3) minutes to prevent (a.stasis b.localized acidemia c.hemoconcentration d.all of the above e.none of the above).

7. Maintain firm pressure at least (a.2 b.3 c.5 d.7) minutes for clients with clotting disorders and those on anticoagulant therapy.

8. Forcing the blood from the syringe into the tube causes (a.hemolysis b.blood viscosity c.hemoconcentration d.none of the above).

9. Shaking the tube with the collected blood specimen will cause (a.hemolysis b.blood viscosity c.hemoconcentration d.none of the above) of red blood cells.

10. Additives in the test tube prevent (a.blood viscosity b.blood clot formation c.hemoconcentration d.none of the above).

11. If client becomes dizzy or faint, position the head lower (a.than the chest b.above the knees c.between knees d.none of the above).

12. Test tubes are pre-warmed when collecting blood specimen for (a.cryoglobulin levels b.ammonia levels c.lactic acid levels d.none of the above).

13. Icing the test tube before delivery to the laboratory is a requirement for an obtained specimen for (a.cryoglobulin levels b.ammonia levels c.lactic acid levels d.none of the above).

14. Tourniquet is never used in collecting blood samples for (a.cryoglobulin levels b.ammonia levels c.lactic acid levels d.vitamin levels).

15. Test tubes are not exposed to light after obtaining blood samples for (a.cryoglobulin levels b.ammonia levels c.lactic acid levels d.vitamin levels).

16. The most common complications from the venipuncture site are (a.hematoma b.venous collapse c.veinous trauma d.none of the above) and infection.

17. Tie the tourniquet (a.5 to 10 cm b.2 to 4 inches c.7 to 12 cm d. 3 to 6 inches e.A & B only f.B & C only g.none of the above) above the area chosen to make the veins dilate.

18..Using the legs for venipuncture may predispose the client to (a.hematoma b.thrombophlebitis c.paresthesia d.none of the above) and infection.

19. Tourniquet may be optional for a client with large, distended and highly visible veins to prevent the occurrence of hematoma (a.true b.false c.maybe d.none of the above).

20. Ask the client to close his fist loosely as needle is inserted and open it as soon as the needle is in the vein. (a.true b.false c.maybe d.none of the above).

Chapter 3 Intravenous Line

Certain types of IV therapy always require venipuncture and an IV line. It is a common practice in accessing the intravascular part of the human body. The IV line enables administration of fluids, electrolytes, medications and blood to the client. It promotes quick recovery, stabilization and effective care.

Equipment/Materials

20 to 22 gauge catheter for adults and 22 to 24 gauge catheter for children
IV solution bag and tubing
Alcohol swabs/antiseptic swabs
IV pole
Gloves
2 x2 gauze dressing
Tourniquet
Tape
Scissor

Procedure

1. Secure the signed consent form.
***A signed consent form enables the nurse to proceed with the procedure.

2. Wash hands.
***Safety precautions prevent infection and transfer of microorganism.

3. Prepare IV solution by initially checking expiration date and appearance or consistency of the solution.
***Checking the IV solution ensures its sterile properties.

4. Open and unroll the tubing.

5. Close the clamp.
***Closing the clamps prevents the IV solution from leaking.

6. Hang the IV solution bag in the IV pole.

7. Spike the IV solution bag with the tip of the tubing.

8. Compress the sides of the drip chamber to fill halfway.

9. Open the roller clamp.

10. Remove protective cap from the end of the tubing.

11. Flush the tubing using the IV solution.

12. Close the roller clamp.

13. Replace cap protector.

14. Explain procedure to the client.
***Explaining the procedure alleviates anxiety

15. Put on gloves.

16. Assess the veins of the site and palpate for a firm rebound sensation.
***Assessment prevents untoward complication and promotes the safety of the client.

17. Tie the tourniquet 5 to 10 cm (2 to 4 inches) above the area chosen to make the veins dilate.

18. Palpate brachial pulse.
***Tight tourniquet impedes arterial blood flow.

19. Clean the site with the alcohol swab in circulation motion from inner to outer. Let it dry.
***Cleaning the site prevents infection.

20. Immobilize the vein by pressing an inch just below the site using the thumb. Draw the skin taut.
***Immobilizing the vein promotes stability and prevents it from moving during needle insertion.

21. Position and insert the needle to the vein at a 15 to 30 degree angle with the bevel of needle in the upward position.
***This angle with bevel pointed upward prevents the puncture of the posterior wall of the vein.

22. Watch for the quick blood return to ensure needle placement.

23. Advance the catheter at least 1/4 inch into the vein.

24. Loosen the stylet and advance the catheter until the hub rests at the venipuncture site.

25. Release or remove the tourniquet.
***Releasing the tourniquet reestablishes venous blood flow.

26. Stabilize the catheter and remove the stylet from the catheter.

27. Connect the IV tubing to the hub of the catheter.

28. Open the roller clamp to start the infusion at a slow rate to keep the vein open.

29. Secure the catheter by placing a tape over the hub and placing a 2 x 2 gauze pad over the insertion site. Finish by taping to secure its attachment.

30. Remove gloves and dispose of other materials.

31. Set the flow rate according to the order.

Determine the hourly rate by dividing the total volume by the total hours.
Example:

An order of 2000 ml D5W over 6 hours.

Solution:
$$\frac{2000}{6} = 333 \text{ ml/hr}$$

Determine the minute rate based on the drop factor of the infusion set.

The following formula can be used:

Drop factor x ml/min = drop per minute

$$\frac{\text{ml/hr x drop factor}}{60 \text{ minute}} = \text{drops per minute}$$

Example: $\frac{150 \text{ ml x 80 drops per ml}}{60 \text{ minutes}} = \frac{12000 \text{ drops}}{60 \text{ minutes}} = 200$ drops per minute

The common complications from an IV line (peripheral) are phlebitis, infiltration, dislodgement, occlusion, hematoma, infection, allergic reaction, circulatory overload and air embolism.

Phlebitis is manifested by tenderness at the proximal area of the venous catheter, redness with puffiness of the vein and elevated temperature. It is managed by removing the venous catheter, using a larger vein and applying warm soaks. Infiltration is manifested by swelling, blanching, discomfort at the insertion site. It is managed by stopping the infusion, using another site, applying warm soaks and elevating affected extremity. Dislodgement requires securely retaping the catheter. Occlusion is manifested by backflow of blood in the tubing and discomfort at insertion site. It is managed by mild flush injection and starting a new line if occlusion persists. Hematoma is manifested by bruising and tenderness at the injection site. It is managed by removing the catheter, applying warm soaks and using another site. Infection is manifested by fever, chills and malaise. It is managed by obtaining a culture from the affected site, administering antibiotic, discontinuing infusion and starting a new line. Allergic reaction is manifested by itching, watery eyes, bronchospasm, rash, edema and anaphylactic reaction. It is managed by stopping the infusion immediately, administering antihistamine, antiinflammatory, steroids, antipyretic and monitoring the client. Circulatory overload is manifested by venous engorgement, respiratory distress, elevated blood pressure, crackles and discomfort. It is managed by elevating the head of the bed, rechecking flow rate, administering oxygen and medications such as diuretics. Air embolism is manifested by hypotension, respiratory distress, weak pulse, unequal breath sounds and loss of consciousness. It is managed by discontinuing the infusion, administering oxygen and positioning the client on the left side in a trendelenburg position to allow the air to enter the right atrium where it will be dispersed by the pulmonary artery.

Chapter 3 Test (IV Line)

I. Multiple Choice
Choose the best answer from the following statements.

1. The hourly rate of an order of 2000 ml D5W over 10 hours is (a.100 b.200 c.150 d.125 e.none of the above).

2. Tie the tourniquet (a.5 to 10 cm b.2 to 4 inches c.7 to 12 cm d. 3 to 6 inches e.A & B only f.B & C only g.none of the above) above the area chosen to make the veins dilate.

3. Position and insert the needle to the vein at a (a.35 to 45 b.15 to 30 c.5 to 15 d.none of the above) degree angle with the bevel of needle in the upward position.

4. Advance the catheter at least (a.1/2 b.1/3 c.1/4 d.none of the above) inch into the vein.

5. Releasing the tourniquet reestablishes (a.venous b.arterial c.capillary d.none of the above) blood flow.

II Enumeration and filling the blanks.

6-14. What are the common complications from an IV line (peripheral)?

15-16. Infiltration is manifested by _____, _____, discomfort at the insertion site.

17-19. Phlebitis is manifested by tenderness at the _____ area of the venous catheter, redness with _____ of the vein and elevated _____.

20-21. Hematoma is manifested by _____ and _____ at the injection site.

22-24. What are the three common symptoms of Infection?

25-29. What are the symptoms of an allergic reaction?

30-33. What are the symptoms of circulatory overload?

34-38. What are the symptoms of air embolism?

39-41. What are the ways of managing Air embolism?

42-44. Managing an air embolism from an IV line includes positioning the client on the _____ side in a trendelenburg position to allow the air to enter the _____ atrium that will be dispersed by the pulmonary _____ .

45-50. What are the ways of managing an Allergic reaction?

51-53. What are the ways of managing.Hematoma?

54-57. What are the ways of managing an infiltration?

58-60. What are the ways of managing a circulatory overload?

Chapter 4 Blood Transfusion

Blood transfusion is a procedure that is used to replenish the volume and oxygenation of the circulatory system by increasing the mass quantity of the circulating red blood cells. It comprises whole blood and packed RBCs (red blood cells). Whole blood transfusion is utilized when there is hemorrhage whereas packed RBCs are used to prevent possible fluid and circulatory overload when there are depressed levels of blood values accompanying normal blood volume.

Equipment/Materials

Blood transfusion set/Y tubing
Whole blood or packed RBC
250 ml of normal saline (0.9% NaCl) solution
IV pole
Protective equipment (gloves, gown, face shield)
IV cannula/venous catheter/vascular access device

Procedure

1. Explain the procedure to the client and make sure that the consent form is signed.
***Explaining the procedure to the client prevents anxiety and enables cooperation. A signed consent form signifies acceptance and understanding of the procedure. The nurse cannot proceed with the transfusion without a signed consent form.

2. Check the patency of the IV cannula or venous catheter including the integrity of the tissue around the site.
***A 16 or 18 gauge cannula is preferred. Patency is verified to ensure optimal infusion. Signs of infiltration and infection will harm the client.

3. Assess vital signs and record it.
***Changes from the baseline vital signs will prompt the nurse regarding transfusion reaction.

4. Obtain whole blood or packed RBCs 30 minutes of the transfusion time.

5. Check the blood bag for expiration date, color, consistency, blood group, Rh compatibility, identification number if present and for abnormal features such as clumping and gas bubbles.
***Two licensed professionals usually perform the checking depending on the facility protocol. This is done to ensure safety of the client, avoid legal problems and prevent untoward complication such as hemolytic reactions.

6. Put on protective equipment for safety and to prevent infection for both nurses and client.

7. Open blood administration kit.

8. Close all clamps on the Y tube set.
***The Y tube provides the ability to switch from infusing normal saline to blood. Closing clamps prevents accidental spillage.

9. Insert line spikes accordingly. Spike the normal saline bag.

10. Hang on IV pole.

11. Open the roller clamp until tubing from normal saline bag is filled.

12. Close the clamp on the unused tubing.

13. Squeeze the drip chamber until it is half full.

14. Open the lower roller clamp to allow normal saline to fill the tubing up to the hub.
***Normal saline maintains venous patency. Priming the tube eliminates air bubbles.

15. Close the clamp.

16. Spike the blood bag. Make sure to invert the blood bag once or twice before spiking.
***Inverting the blood bag distributes the blood cells equally to prevent clumping and blood clotting.

17. Hang on IV pole.

18. Open clamp on the inlet tube to allow blood to fill the filter completely.

19. Close the lower clamp.

20. Attach the tubing to the IV cannula or venous catheter or another venous access device.

21. Infuse the blood at a flow rate no greater than 5 ml for the first 15 minutes then observe for signs of transfusion reaction.
***Gradual infusion enables the nurse to observe for untoward reaction.

22. Adjust flow rate according to the physician's order.

23. Clear IV line with normal saline after blood has infused.
***Normal saline flushes the IV line maintaining its potency.

24. Appropriately dispose blood bag and other equipment according to the protocols of the facility.
***Proper disposal reduces transmission of microorganism.

25. Monitor IV site for status of infusion and vital signs.
***Monitoring prevents untoward complications such as infiltration, phlebitis and transfusion reaction.

The common unexpected outcomes from blood transfusion are transfusion reaction, infiltration, phlebitis and fluid overload. Transfusion reaction is manifested with symptoms such as fever, chills, tachycardia, tachypnea, wheezing, dyspnea, headache, flushing, hives, hypotension and gastrointestinal disturbances. The transfusion is immediately stopped and disconnected when transfusion reaction occurs, and vein is kept open with slow infusion of normal saline. Phlebitis and infiltration is managed by inserting a new IV cannula or vascular access device on another site. Fluid overload is manifested with symptoms of dyspnea and crackles. The transfusion is either stopped or slowed and the client's head is elevated. Physician is always informed if any unexpected outcome occurs.

Chapter 4 Test (Blood Transfusion)

I. Multiple Choice
Choose the best answer from the following statements.

1. Obtain whole blood or packed RBCs (a.10 b.20 c.30 d.40) minutes of the transfusion time.

2. Changes from the baseline vital signs will prompt the nurse regarding (a.transfusion reaction b.infiltration c.hematoma d.hemoconcentration e.none of the above).

3. (a.one b.two c.three d.none of the above) licensed professionals usually perform the checking depending on the facility protocol.

4. Priming the tube eliminates (a.patency b.viscosity c.air bubbles d.none of the above).

5. The Y tube provides the ability to switch from infusing (a.normal saline b.medication c.TPN d.none of the above) to blood.

6. Normal saline maintains venous (a.viscosity b.patency c.alkalinity d.none of the above).

7. Inverting the blood bag distributes the blood cells equally to prevent (a.clumping b.acidemia c.chilling d.none of the above) and blood clotting.

8-10. Infuse the blood at a flow rate no greater than (a.10 b.7 c.5 d.3) ml for the first (a.15 b.20 c.30 d.10) minutes and observe for (a.hematoma b.infiltration c.hemoconcentration d.transfusion reaction).

II. Enumeration

11-20. What are the symptoms of a transfusion reaction during a blood transfusion?

Chapter 5 Intradermal Injection

Intradermal injection is primarily done for skin testing such as in allergy testing and screening for tuberculin using a PPD (purified protein derivative) solution. The effect is local rather than systemic. The forearm and upper back are common sites for intradermal injection.

Equipment/Materials

1 ml tuberculin syringe with PPD solution
25 to 27 gauge needle
Alcohol swabs
Gloves

Procedure

1.Explain the procedure to the client and make sure that the consent form is signed if needed.
***Explaining the procedure to the client prevents anxiety and enables cooperation. A signed consent form if needed signifies acceptance and understanding of the procedure. The nurse can not proceed with the procedure without a signed consent form in some instances.

2.Prepare the syringe and needle with PPD solution.
***Preparing the solution prior to injection conserves time and effort.

3.Wash hands and put on gloves.

***Safety precautions prevent the spread of microorganisms.

4.Inspect injection site for bruises, swelling and obvious deformities.
***Injection site should be clear for accuracy in interpreting results.

5.The injection site in the forearm should be 3 to 4 fingerwidths below the antecubital space.

6.Clean the site with alcohol swab in circular motion from inner to outer aspect from the site.

7.Pull the cap from the needle of the syringe.

8.Stretch the skin over the site by using the thumb and forefinger of the non-dominant hand.

9.Insert the needle slowly at 5 to 15 degree angle with bevel pointed upward.

10.Advance at least 1/8 inch below the skin with the tip of the needle seen through the skin surface.

11. Slowly inject the PPD solution until a small wheal or bleb is formed under the skin surface.
***The formation of a wheal or bleb indicates the deposition of the medication in the dermal area of the skin.

12. Withdraw the needle while applying gentle pressure with an alcohol swab.

13. The site is never massaged to prevent dispersing the medication into surrounding tissue.

14. Discard needle, syringe and gloves in their appropriate containers.
***Discarding the needle in the sharps container prevents accidental prick.

Chapter 5 Test (Intradermal Injection)

I. Fill in the blanks with the appropriate answer.

1-2. Intradermal injection is primarily done for _____ such as in allergy testing and screening for tuberculin using a PPD _____ solution.

3-4. Preparing the syringe with solution prior to the injection conserves _____ and _____..

5-6. The injection site in the forearm should be 3 to 4 _____ below the _____.

7-8. Stretch the skin over the site by using the _____ and _____ of the non-dominant hand.

9-10. Insert the needle slowly at _____ degree angle with bevel pointed _____.

11-12. Advance the needle at least _____ inch below the skin with the tip of the needle seen through the _____.

13-15. The formation of a _____ or _____ indicates the deposition of the medication in the _____ area of the skin.

Chapter 6 Subcutaneous Injection

Subcutaneous injection is used primarily to administer a medication that is absorbed gradually into the loose connective tissues below the dermal layer of the skin. The most common medications that are administered subcutaneously are insulin, tetanus toxoid, allergy medications, epinephrine and vitamin B 12. These medications are water soluble, isotonic, non-viscous and non-irritating. The common sites for subcutaneous injections are the abdomen, outer aspect of the upper arm and the anterior aspect of the thigh. Rotation of injection site is important to prevent lipodystrophy.

Equipment/Materials

1 to 3 ml syringe
Vial of medication
25 to 27 gauge needle
Alcohol swabs
Gloves

Procedure

1. Explain the procedure to the client and make sure that the consent form is signed if needed. ***Explaining the procedure to the client prevents anxiety and enables cooperation. A signed consent form if needed signifies acceptance and understanding of the procedure. The nurse cannot proceed with the injection without a signed consent form in some instances.

2. Wash hands.

3. Prepare the syringe and needle with the vial of medication.

4. Remove the cap of the vial and wipe off the rubber seal with alcohol swab

5. Pick up syringe and needle. Put them together and turn tightly enough to prevent detachment during the procedure.

6. Remove the cap of the needle.

7. Pull back the plunger and draw an amount of air that is equivalent to the amount of medication that will be aspirated in the vial.

8. Insert the tip of the needle through the center of the vial that lies on flat surface.

9. Inject the drawn air into the vial.

10. Pick up both vial and syringe and invert the vial upwards while holding firmly onto the syringe at your eye level.

11. The tip of the needle inside the vial should be below the fluid level. Adjust if needed.

12. Pull plunger to allow air pressure and medication to fill the syringe to the desired amount.

13. Dislodge any air bubbles by tapping the side of the syringe until the air bubble goes up and emerges from the fluid.

14. Position the tip of the needle above the fluid level inside the syringe and eject the air.

15. Remove the needle from the vial by pulling the barrel of the syringe.

16. Check the amount of medication in the syringe at eye level.

17. Needle may be recapped by pointing the needle in the middle of the cap and closed in depending on the facility policy.
***Preparing the medication prior to injection conserves time and effort.

18. Put on gloves.
***Safety precaution prevents the spread of microorganism.

19. Position the client in a sitting position.

20. Inspect injection site for bruises, swelling and obvious deformities.
***Injection site should be clear of abnormalities for the safety of the client and for the absorption of the medication.

21. Clean the site with alcohol swab in circulation motion from inner to outer aspect from the site.

22. Pull the cap from the needle of the syringe.

23. Pinch the skin with the non-dominant hand to elevate the subcutaneous tissue.

24. Hold the syringe like a dart at a 45 to 90 degree angle.

25. Inject the needle of the syringe.

26. Release the skin and grasp the lower end of the syringe with the non-dominant hand.

27. Hold the end of the plunger with the dominant hand and pull back the plunger.
***Pulling back the plunger will check for blood visible when a vein is hit by the needle. Presence of blood in the syringe requires restarting a new injection site. Aspiration is contraindicated in certain medications.

28. Slowly administer the medication.

29. Withdraw the needle while applying gentle pressure with an alcohol swab.

30. The site is massaged gently depending on the type of administered medication. Certain medications are not massaged.
***Massaging the injection site promotes distribution and absorption of the medication.

31. Discard needle, syringe and gloves in their appropriate containers.
***Discarding the needle in the sharps container prevents accidental prick.

Chapter 6 Test (Subcutaneous Injection)

I. Multiple Choice
Choose the best answer from the following statements.

1. Subcutaneous injection is used primarily to administer a medication that is absorbed gradually into the (a.loose connective tissues b.compact connective tissue c.muscles d.none of the above) below the dermal layer of the skin.

2. Rotation of injection is important to prevent (a.hematoma b.infection c.lipodystrophy d.none of the above).

3. A (a. 10 to 20 b.25 to 27 c.15 to 20 d.none of the above) gauge needle is ideal for a subcutaneous injection.

4. Pull back the plunger and draw an amount of air that is (a.equivalent b.more c.less d.none of the above) to the amount of medication that will be aspirated in the vial.

5. Insert the tip of the needle through the (a.side b.center c.left side d.right side) of the vial that lies on flat surface.

6. Pick up both vial and syringe and invert the vial (a.down b.sideways c.up d.none of the above) while holding firmly onto the syringe within eye level.

7. The tip of the needle inside the vial should be (a.below b.above c.outside d.none of the above) the fluid level.

8. Dislodge any air bubbles in the syringe by tapping the (a.upper part b.lower part c.side d.none of the above) of syringe until it goes up.

9. Position the tip of the needle (a.below b.above c.sideways d.none of the above) the fluid level inside the syringe and eject the air.

10. Hold the syringe like a dart at a (a.15 to 20 b. 25 to 30 c. 30 to 35 d.45 to 90) degree angle and inject the needle of the syringe.

II. Enumeration

11-15. What are the most common medications administered subcutaneously?

16-19. What are the characteristic of a subcutaneous medications?

20-22. What are the common sites for subcutaneous injections?

Chapter 7 Intramuscular Injection

Intramuscular injection is administered to enable quick absorption of medication in the deep muscle tissues. The most common site for intramuscular injections are deltoid muscle, vastus lateralis muscle, ventrogluteal muscle and dorsogluteal muscle. Vastus lateralis muscle is located on the anterior lateral aspect of the thigh. Dorsogluteal muscle is located in the upper outer quadrant of the buttocks. Deltoid muscle is located in the upper arm.

Equipments/Materials

1 to 3 ml syringe
Vial of medication
19 to 23 gauge needle
Alcohol swabs
Gloves

Procedure

1. Explain the procedure to the client and make sure that the consent form is signed if needed. ***Explaining the procedure to the client deters anxiety and enables cooperation. A signed consent form if needed signifies acceptance and understanding of the procedure. The nurse cannot proceed with the injection without a signed consent form in some instances.

2. Wash hands.

3. Prepare the syringe and needle with the vial of medication.

4. Remove the cap of the vial and wipe off the rubber seal with alcohol swab.

5. Pick up syringe and needle. Put together and turn tight enough to lock or prevent from being detached during the procedure.

6. Remove the cap of the needle.

7. Pull back the plunger and draw an amount of air that is equivalent to the amount of medication that will be aspirated in the vial.

8. Insert the tip of the needle through the center of the vial that lies on flat surface.

9. Inject the drawn air into the vial.

10. Pick up both vial and syringe and invert the vial upwards while holding firmly onto the syringe within eye level.

11. The tip of the needle inside the vial should be below the fluid level.

12. Pull plunger to allow air pressure and medication to fill the syringe up to desired amount.

13. Dislodge any air bubbles by tapping the side of syringe until it goes up and emerges from the fluid.

14. Position the tip of the needle above the fluid level inside the syringe and eject the air.

15. Remove the needle from the vial by pulling the barrel of the syringe.

16. Check the amount of medication in the syringe at eye level.

17. Needle may be recapped by pointing it in the middle of the cap and closing it depending on the facility policy.
***Preparing the solution prior to injection conserves time and effort.

18. Put on gloves.
***Safety precaution prevents the spread of microorganism.

19. Position the client according to the site of injection.
The client will lie supine with the knee slightly flexed if the chosen site is the vastus lateralis muscle. Position the client on the side or back with the knee and hip slightly flexed if the chosen site is the ventrogluteal muscle. The client is positioned prone with feet on side with the upper knee and hip flexed and placed in front of the lower leg if the chosen site is the dorsogluteal muscle. Position the client sitting if the chosen site is deltoid muscle.
***Positioning the client appropriately will promote relaxation and minimizes discomfort.

20. Inspect injection site for bruises, swelling and obvious deformities.
***Injection site should be clear of abnormalities for the safety of the client and for the absorption of the medication.

21. Clean the site with alcohol swab in circulation motion from inner to outer aspect from the site.

22. Pull the cap from the needle of the syringe.

23. Pinch a large section of the site or spread the skin tightly as possible.

24. Hold the syringe like a dart at a 90 degree angle and inject the needle of the syringe.

25. Release the skin and grasp the lower end of the syringe with the non-dominant hand.

26. Hold the end of the plunger with the dominant hand and pull back the plunger.
***Pulling back the plunger will check for blood that occurs when a vein is hit by the needle. Presence of blood in the syringe requires restarting a new injection site.

27. Slowly administer the medication.

28. Withdraw the needle while applying gentle pressure with an alcohol swab.

29. The site is massaged gently depending on the type of administered medication.
***Massaging the injection site promotes distribution and absorption of the medication.

30. Discard needle, syringe and gloves in their appropriate containers.
***Discarding the needle in the sharps container prevents accidental pricks.

Chapter 7 Test (Intramuscular Injection)

I. Multiple Choice
Choose the best answer from the following statements.

1. Intramuscular injection is administered to enable (a.gradual b.slow c.quick d.none of the above) absorption of medication in the deep muscle tissues.

2. (a.Dorsogluteal b.Deltoid c.Ventrogluteal d.Vastus lateralis) muscle is located on the anterior lateral aspect of the thigh.

3. (a.Dorsogluteal b.Deltoid c.Ventrogluteal d.Vastus lateralis) muscle is located in the upper outer quadrant of the buttocks.

4. (a.Dorsogluteal b.Deltoid c.Ventrogluteal d.Vastus lateralis) muscle is located in the upper arm.

5. The client will lie supine with the knee slightly flexed if the chosen site is the (a.dorsogluteal b.deltoid c.ventrogluteal d.vastus lateralis) muscle.

6. Position the client on the side or back with the knee and hip slightly flexed if the chosen site is the (a.dorsogluteal b.deltoid c.ventrogluteal d.vastus lateralis) muscle.

7. The client is positioned prone with feet on side with the upper knee and hip flexed and placed in front of the lower leg if the chosen site is the (a.dorsogluteal b.deltoid c.ventrogluteal d.vastus lateralis) muscle.

8. Position the client sitting if the chosen site is (a.dorsogluteal b.deltoid c.ventrogluteal d.vastus lateralis) muscle.

9. Clean the site with alcohol swab in circular motion from (a.inner to outer b.outer to inner c.center downward d.upward to downward) aspect from the site.

10-11. Pinch a (a.small b.large c.central d.none of the above) section of the site or spread the skin (a.loosely b.gradually c.tightly d.none of the above) as possible when performing the intramuscular injection on the chosen site.

12. Hold the syringe like a dart at (a.90 b.30 to 45 c.60 d.none of the above) degree angle and inject the needle of the syringe.

13. Pulling back the plunger will check for (a.air b.blood c.medication d.none of the above) that occurs when a vein is hit by the needle.

14. Massaging the injection site promotes distribution and (a.expansion b.expulsion c.absorption d.none of the above) of the medication.

15. Presence of blood in the syringe requires (a.starting b.pushing c.continuing d.none of the above) an injection site.

16. The commonly used gauge of needle for intramuscular injection is from (a.25 to 27 b.19 to 23 c.25 to 30 d.30 to 35 e.none of the above).

II. Enumeration

17-20. What are the most common sites for intramuscular injections?

21-25. What are the common items of equipment utilized in an intramuscular injection?

Answer Key

Chapter 1(Overview of Anatomy and Physiology)

The Muscular System

I. Multiple Choice Choose the best answer/s from the following statements. There could be one or more answer/s from the selection

1. A   Abduction is a movement away from the midline plane of the body.

2. B   Adduction is a movement toward the midline plane of the body.

3. C   Dorsiflexion is a movement where the foot is brought closer to the shin upward.

4. D   Extension is a movement of increasing the angle between two surfaces such as straightening the limbs of the body.

5. A   Flexion is a movement that decreases the angle between two surfaces such as bending a limb of the body.

6. B   Plantar flexion is a movement that extends the foot downwards.

7. C   Pronation is a movement where the palm is turned backward and down.

8. D   Rotation is a movement where there is circular movement around an axis.

9. A   Supination is a movement where the palm is turned forward and up.

10. B   Ligament is a fibrous connective tissue that connects a bone to another bone in the body.

11. C   Tendon is a fibrous connective tissue that connects a muscle to a bone.

12. D   Bursa (ber-sa) is a fluid filled sac that is lined by a synovial membrane that provides cushioning between muscles and bones in a joint.

13. A   Fascia (fash-e-a) is a fibrinous membrane or a connective tissue that separates and surrounds muscles.

14. B   The striated muscle is also called a skeletal muscle. It functions voluntarily and is consciously manipulated.

15. C   The smooth muscle is located in the internal organs of the human body. It is also called visceral muscle. It reacts involuntary and is not controlled consciously.

The Cardiovascular System

I. Multiple Choice.   Choose the best answer/s from the following statements. There could be one or more answer/s from the selection.

1. D   Atrium (ai-tre-um) is the upper chamber of the heart where the blood enters.

2. B   Ventricle (ven-tri-kl) is the lower chamber of the heart where the blood is collected and pushed out.

3. C   Tricuspid valve (trai-kus-pid valv) is a valve consisting of three flaps. It is located between the right atrium and right ventricle. It is also called the right atrioventricular valve.

4. A   Pulmonary valve (pul-mo-ner-e valv) is a valve consisting of three cusps. It is located between the right ventricle and pulmonary artery.

5. D   Mitral valve (mai-tral valv) is a valve with two flaps. It is located between the left atrium and the left ventricle. It is also called bicuspid valve or left atrioventricular valve.

6. B   Aortic valve (ai-or-tik valv) is a valve that has three leaflets. It is located between the left ventricle and the aorta.

7. C   Myocardium (mai-o-kar-de-um) is the middle layer of the heart consisting of cardiac muscles.

8. A   Pericardium (per-i-kar-de-um) is the outermost layer of the heart consisting of a double layered membrane that covers the heart.

9. D   Sinoatrial node (sai-no-ae-tre-al nod) is a tissue that generates impulses. It is located in the right atrium of the heart. It is also called the pacemaker of the heart.

10. B   Atrioventricular node (ae-tre-o-ven-trik-u-lar nod) is a tissue that coordinates impulses between the atrium and the ventricle. It is located between the atria and ventricles of the heart.

11. C   Bundle of His (bun-dl of his) is tissue that transmits impulses from the atrioventricular node to the Purkinje fibers.

12. A   Purkinje fiber is a fiber that generates electrical impulses to the ventricle. It is located in the inner ventricular walls of the heart.

13. D   Diastole (dai-as-to-le) is a period when the heart refills with blood and the ventricles are relaxing.

14. B   Systole (sis-to-le) is a period when the ventricle of the heart is contracting.

15. C   Vasoconstriction (vaz-o-kon-strik-shun) is the narrowing of a blood vessel due to the contraction of its muscles.

The Hematological System

I.   Matching type. Match column A with column B. There could be one or more answer/s from the selection.

C, D   1. Blood type AB

A   2. Blood type O

B, G   3. Blood type B

E, F   4. Blood type A

Blood type AB is a universal receiver. This blood type cannot donate to blood types A and B because of its antigens. Blood type O is known as the universal donor because it can be donated to all blood types but can only receive its own blood type. Blood type B can receive blood from types B and O but can only donate to types AB and B. Finally blood type A can receive blood from types A and O but can only donate to types AB and A.

II. Multiple Choice   Choose the appropriate word/s to complete the following statements. There could be one or more answer/s from the selection.

ABC   1. Agranulocytes (ai-gran-u-lo-saits) are white blood cells with one large nucleus. They comprise the lymphocytes and monocytes.

A   2. Erythrocyte (e-rith-ro-sait) is a red blood cell.

B   3. Granulocytes (gran-u-lo-saits) are white blood cells with multiple granules. They form the basophils, eosinophils and neutrophils.

B   4. Leukocyte (loo-ko-sait) is a white blood cell.

D   5. Thrombocyte (throm-bo-sait) is a platelet cell.

A   6. Basophil (ba-so-fil) is a type of white blood cell with large and dark granules.

C   7. Eosinophil (e-o-sin-o-fil) is a type of white blood cell with dense and reddish granules.

C   8. Lymphocyte (lim-fo-sait) is a type of white blood cell with large dark staining nucleus. These cells produce antibodies.

D   9. Monocyte (mon-o-sait) is a type of white blood cell that is formed in the bone marrow. It becomes a macrophage after leaving the blood. It functions for phagocytosis.

A   10. Neutrophil (nu-tro-fil) is a type of white blood cell with neutral staining granules. It is produced in the bone marrow and functions for phagocytosis.

Chapter 2 Venipuncture

I. Multiple Choice

1. A
2. B
3. A
4. B
5. C
6. D

8.A
9.A
10.B
11.C
12.A
13.B
14.C
15.D
16.A
17.E
18.B
19.A
20.A

Chapter 3 IV Line

I. Multiple Choice

1.B
2.E
3.B
4.C
5.A

II Enumeration and filling the blanks.

6-14. phlebitis, infiltration, dislodgement, occlusion, hematoma, infection, allergic reaction, circulatory overload and air embolism

15. swelling

16. blanching

17. proximal

18. puffiness

19. temperature

20. bruising

21. tenderness

22-24. fever, chills and malaise.

25-29. itching, watery eyes, bronchospasm, rash, edema and anaphylactic reaction

30-33. venous engorgement, respiratory distress, elevated blood pressure, crackles and discomfort.

34-38. hypotension, respiratory distress, weak pulse, unequal breath sounds and loss of consciousness.

39-41. discontinuing the infusion, administering oxygen and positioning the client on the left side in a trendelenburg position to allow air to enter the right atrium that will be dispersed by the pulmonary artery.

42. left

43. right

44. artery

45-50. stopping the infusion immediately, administering antihistamine, antiinflammatory, steroids, antipyretic and monitoring the client.

51-53. removing the catheter, applying warm soaks and using another site.

54-57. stopping the infusion, using another site, applying warm soaks and elevating the affected extremity.

58-60. elevating the head of the bed, rechecking flow rate, administering oxygen and medications such as diuretics.

Chapter 4 Blood Transfusion

I. Multiple Choice

1. C
2. A
3. B
4. C
5. A
6. B
7. A
8. C
9. A
10. D

II. Enumeration

11-20. fever, chills, tachycardia, tachypnea, wheezing, dyspnea, headache, flushing, hives, hypotension and gastrointestinal disturbances

Chapter 5 Intradermal Injection

1. skin testing

2. purified protein derivative

3. time

4. effort

5. 3 to 4 finger widths

6. antecubital space

7. thumb

8. forefinger

9. 5 to 15

10. upward

11. 1/8

12. skin surface

13. wheal

14. bleb

15. dermal

Chapter 6 Subcutaneous Injection

I. Multiple Choice

1. A
2. C
3. B

4.A
5.B
6.C
7.A
8.C
9.B
10.D

II. Enumeration

1-15. insulin, tetanus toxoid, allergy medications, epinephrine and vitamin B 12

16-19. water soluble, isotonic, nonviscous and non-irritating

20-22. abdomen, outer aspect of the upper arm and the anterior aspect of the thigh.

Chapter 7 Intramuscular Injection

I. Multiple Choice

1.C
2.D
3.A
4.B
5.D
6.C
7.A
8.B
9.A
10.B
11.C
12.A
13.B
14.C
15.A
16.B

II. Enumeration

17-20. deltoid muscle, vastus lateralis muscle, ventrogluteal muscle and dorso lateral muscle.

21-25. 1 to 3 ml syringe, vial of medication, 19 to 23 gauge needle, alcohol swabs, gloves and sharps container.

References

I would like to express my gratitude to:

Dr. Lee Robbins for his support in writing this book.

Anatomy and Physiology, Wiley and Sons, New Jersey, 2007
Fundamentals of Nursing 7th Edition, Mosby, Canada, 2009
Medical – Surgical Nursing 4th Edition, Prentice Hall, New Jersey, 2008
Nursing Assistants, Mosby, Philadelphia, 2004
Pathophysiology of Disease 2nd Edition, Appleton and Lange, 1997
Pharmacology in Nursing 21st Edition, Mosby, Missouri 2001
The Johns Hopkins Consumer Guide to Medical Tests, Medletter Associates Inc, New York, 2001
Wikipidea Free Internet Dictionary

Connect with me online :

Facebook: http://www.facebook.com/solomon.barroa
Twitter: https://twitter.com/solomonbarroa
Amazon: amazon.com/author/solomonbarroa
LinkedIn: http://www.linkedin.com/in/solomonbarroa

Index

air, 6, 23, 28, 34, 35, 38, 39
air bubbles, 28, 35, 39
alcohol pad, 17
allergy testing, 31
angle, 10, 17, 22, 31, 35
anxiety, 22, 27, 31, 34, 38
aseptic technique, 18
bevel, 17, 22, 31
bleb, 32
blood, 4, 6, 7, 8, 9, 16, 17, 18, 21, 22, 23, 27, 28, 29, 35, 39
blood sample, 16
Blood transfusion, 27
blood types, 8
bruises, 31, 35, 39
cap, 22, 31, 34, 35, 38, 39
cardiovascular system, 6
catheter, 21, 22, 23, 27, 28
clamp, 21, 22, 23, 28
collection tubes, 16
consent form, 21, 27, 31, 34, 38
deltoid muscle, 38, 39
dermis, 9
diagnostic studies, 16
dislodgement, 23
dorso gluteal muscle, 39
drip chamber, 21, 28
drop factor, 23
drops per minute, 23
epidermis, 9
extravasation, 18
facility protocol, 27
forearm, 16, 31
Fundamentals of Nursing, 51
gauge needle, 16, 31, 34, 38
gauze pad, 17, 23
gauze pads, 16
gloves, 16, 18, 22, 23, 27, 31, 32, 35, 36, 39, 40
heart, 6, 7, 9
hematoma, 16, 17, 18, 23
hemoconcentration, 17, 18
hemolysis, 17, 18
hourly rate, 23
hypodermis, 9
infection, 16, 18, 21, 22, 23, 27
infiltration, 23, 27, 29
insulin, 34
integumentary system, 9
Intradermal injection, 31
Intramuscular injection, 38
IV cannula, 27, 28, 29
IV line, 21, 23, 28
IV pole, 21, 27, 28
IV solution, 21, 22
laboratory, 4, 18
massage, 32, 36, 40
medication, 32, 34, 35, 36, 38, 39, 40
muscles, 9, 10
needle, 16, 17, 18, 22, 31, 32, 34, 35, 36, 38, 39, 40
normal saline, 27, 28, 29
oxygenated blood, 6
packed RBCs, 27
patency, 27, 28
phlebitis, 23, 29
plunger, 17, 34, 35, 38, 39
PPD (purified protein derivative), 31
pressure, 6, 7, 8, 17, 24, 32, 35, 36, 39, 40
procedure, 4, 16, 21, 22, 27, 31, 34, 38
sharps container, 32, 36, 40
site, 16, 17, 18, 22, 23, 27, 29, 31, 32, 35, 36, 38, 39, 40
Skeletal muscles, 9
skin, 8, 9, 17, 22, 31, 32, 34, 35, 39
Subcutaneous injection, 34
syringe, 16, 17, 18, 31, 32, 34, 35, 36, 38, 39, 40
tape, 16, 23
thrombophlebitis, 16
tourniquet, 16, 17, 22
transfusion reaction, 27, 28, 29
tube, 16, 17, 18, 28
tuberculin syringe, 31

tubing, 21, 22, 23, 28
Vacutainer tubes, 16
vastus lateralis muscle, 38, 39
vein, 6, 16, 17, 22, 23, 29, 35, 39
veins, 6, 7, 16, 22
Venipuncture, 1, 16
venous catheter, 23, 27
ventrogluteal muscle, 38, 39
vial, 34, 35, 38, 39
vital signs, 27, 29
wheal, 32
whole blood, 27
Y tube, 28
Y tubing, 27

***Kindly write a review about this book for Amazon or other sites to help other readers that could benefit from this text. Thank you.

And please feel free to browse my other books @ Amazon.com

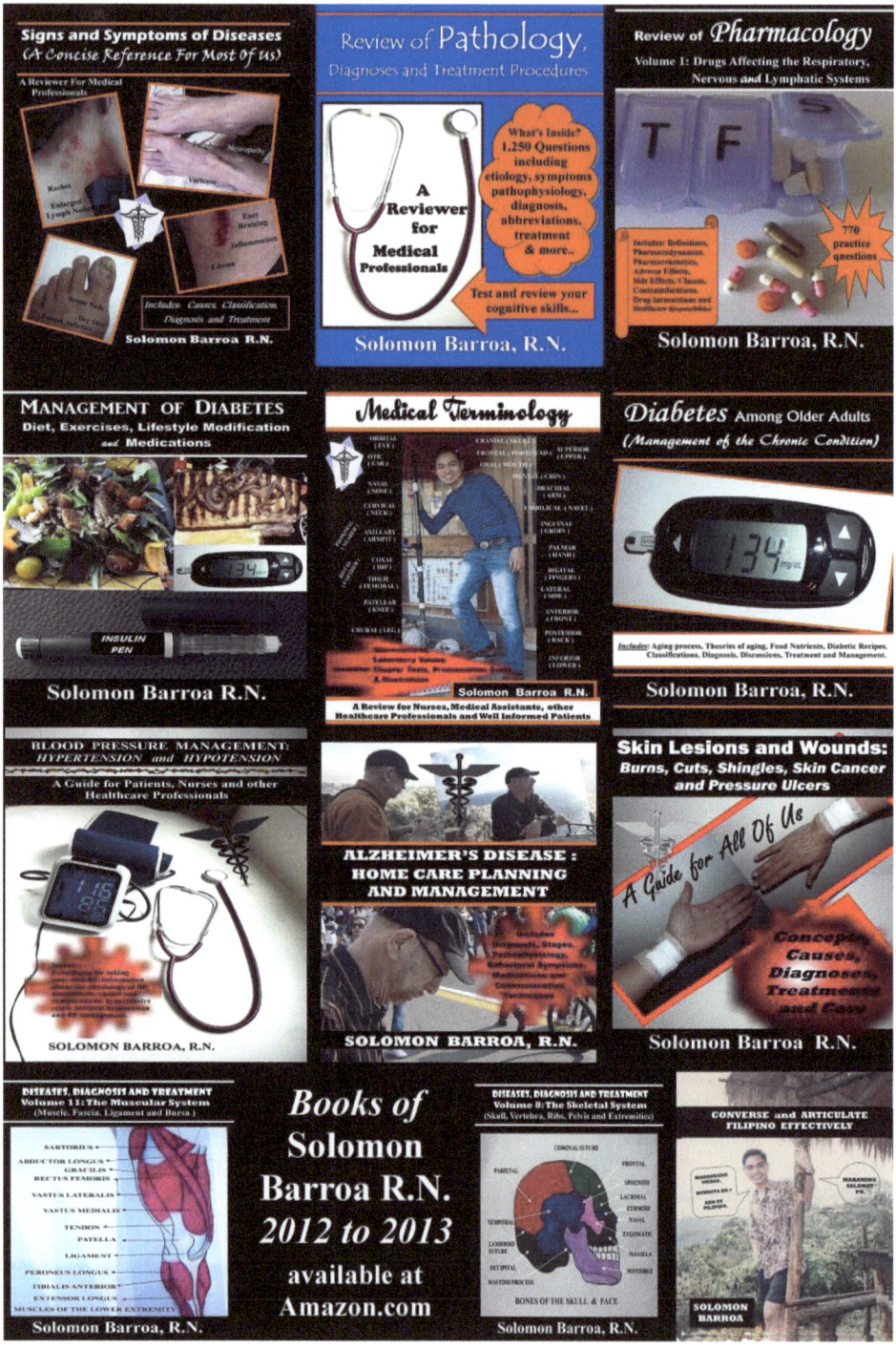

www.ingramcontent.com/pod-product-compliance
Lightning Source LLC
Chambersburg PA
CBHW040743200526
45159CB00023B/1652